Secrets of Growth Hormone

To Build Muscle Mass
Increase Bone Density
And Burn Body Fat!

Turn back the aging clock by learning how to restore your Growth Hormone to youthful levels.

Look great!
Feel great!
Lose weight!
Have better sex!

Y.L. Wright, M.A.
LULU.COM

First Edition

Copyright © 2011 by Y.L. Wright, M.A.

All Rights Reserved. No part of this document may be reproduced without written consent from the author.

ISBN 978-1-105-09213-8

Published by Lulu.com in the United States

Printed in the United States of America

MEDICAL DISCLAIMER:

The following text is for general information only. It contains the opinions and ideas of the author. Careful attention has been paid to insure the accuracy of the information, but the author and the publisher cannot assume responsibility for the validity or consequences of its use. The intention of this book is to provide helpful information. This information is not intended to diagnose or treat any disease. This book is sold with the understanding that the author and publisher are not rendering medical, health, or any other professional services. See your medical or health professional concerning any health concerns or before following any suggestions made in this book or drawing inferences from it. The author and publisher specifically disclaim all responsibility for any liability, loss, or risk incurred as a direct or indirect consequence of using this book's contents. Any use of the information found in this book is the sole responsibility of the reader. Any dietary, nutrient, hormone, and medication suggestions found in this book are to be followed only under the supervision of a medical doctor or other endocrine specialist. Any reference to particular companies or supplements is only for the benefit of the reader. The author receives no compensation from endorsement of any product.

ACKNOWLEDGMENTS:

This book is written for you. If even one person finds their way out of chronic disease and suffering into health, it has been worth it.

TABLE OF CONTENTS

Introduction **3**

1. **What Does Growth Hormone Do?** **6**
2. **Growth Hormone Decreases as We Age** ... **7**
3. **What are the Symptoms of Adult GH Deficiency (AGHD)?** **8**
4. **Most Physicians Won't Treat GH Levels That Aren't Really, Really Low** **9**
5. **Subclinical GH May Be Confused with Other Hormone Deficiencies** **12**
6. **Why Treat GH Deficiency/Subclinical Depression/Suboptimal GH Levels?** **13**
7. **GH Interacts with Every Other Hormone** ... **15**
8. **How Do You Know if Your Own Levels of Growth Hormone are Inadequate?** **16**
9. **Before You Begin Treatment** **18**
10. **How Can I Raise my GH Naturally?** **20**
11. **Treatment** **23**

12. Treatment Modalities 24

1. Hypothalamic peptides & GH stimulants ... 24
Symbiotropin®
Meditropin®

2. Injectable secretagogues 25
GH-releasing peptides-6 (GHRP-6)
Hexarelin

3. GHRH injections 26
Sermorelin

4. Injectable Human Growth Hormone (HGH) .. 27
HGHr

5. Long-chain IGF-1 injections 29
Increlix

6. Tissue Growth factors 29

References 30

Index 33

Introduction

GROWTH HORMONE (GH) IS A HOT TOPIC.

It seems that all of the movie stars, celebrities, and bodybuilders are taking it, and they look fantastic. Baby boomers interested in anti-aging are taking it and saying that it keeps them young.

But you may have heard that it is expensive... and dangerous. So what's the story? What are *your* options? Do you need it? Should you take it? How do you use it? Can you afford it? Let's have a look.

Human Growth Hormone (HGH) is a very important hormone that should not be overlooked by anyone who is interested in living a long and healthy life.

Please carefully read this book before making any decisions about using GH supplements. This book could save you from an early death, either from using risky supplements or from not doing anything at all.

We will look first at the function of GH in the body. Then we will see how GH levels drop as we get older, when to intervene, and what treatment options are available to optimize health.

You will learn about the symptoms of Adult GH Deficiency (AGHD) to determine if you may be a candidate for replacement. Then you will find out how to get tested and what tests you will need.

Before you begin treatment, *there are some things you must know.*

- We will discuss the risks of GH supplementation.

- We will also address the importance of maintaining adequate DHEA levels.

- We will see how toxicity from the environment may cause insensitivity to the GH that your body *is* making.

- Also before beginning treatment, we will explore ways to raise your body's own GH production by changing your diet and exercise routine.

- Beneficial, yet harmless supplements will be recommended.

- We will look specifically at how GH production in the body is stimulated (or suppressed).

- We will present more ways that you can influence your GH levels.

- We will discuss the strict legal environment surrounding the prescription of HGH and GHRH (treatments for AGHD).

- You will learn how to find one of the few doctors who will treat the GH decline associated with aging.

- We will also define the difference between Adult GH Deficiency (AGHD), subclinically low GH levels, and suboptimal GH insufficiency, an important distinction that determines how difficult it is to get a prescription.

Next we will get to the really good part—the part of the book you have all been waiting for. What are the specific treatment modalities for GH deficiency?

Exactly what supplements can I take that will increase my own GH? Where can I get them? How safe is each of them and how much do they cost?

What side effects can result from using these products, especially HGH injections? What are the contraindications? Who should not take these supplements under any circumstances? Let's find out.

1. What Does Growth Hormone Do?

GROWTH HORMONE (GH), as denoted by its name, stimulates the body to grow. However, when the bones *stop* growing (the epiphyses close), GH continues to have profoundly important functions. Call it repair hormone.

If pathologically high levels of GH persist after the bones stop growing, soft tissues and organs in the jaw continue to grow. This is called acromegaly. This is why the giants we see on TV have really big jaws.

GH deficiency causes frailty syndrome, where the body withers. This condition is what we are looking at in this book. If GH *fails* after the bones stop growing, frailty syndrome develops, where the entire body withers. It is like an adult failure to thrive.

The body cannot repair itself properly and goes downhill health-wise. Mild forms of this are common, especially as we get older, but are not often considered by most physicians. MD's traditionally diagnose and treat only extreme hormonal disorders (acromegaly or marked frailty syndrome). Anti-aging physicians treat mild or moderate hormonal dysfunctions before these dysfunctions get extreme.

Let's see what happens to GH as we get older.

2. Growth Hormone Decreases as We Age.

GH drops as we get older and drops significantly with the onset of menopause in women and andropause in men.

In both men and women, GH decreases with age beginning after the early 30's.

GH declines with age (averaging approximately 14% per decade). By 60 years of age, the individual with moderate dysfunction often has only 25% of the GH he or she had at 20.

The decline of GH with age is directly related to many of the symptoms of aging.

GH deficiency contributes to earlier death.[1] Drop in GH causes decreased bone mass and density, decreased muscle mass, and increased fat by up to 40%. It also causes shrinkage in kidneys, stomach, small intestine, liver, and spleen with decreased immune resilience.

Next, let's examine those symptoms of GH decline as we age and find out why most physicians are reluctant to treat those symptoms if the GH decline isn't severe enough to meet their extreme definition of AGHD deficiency.

3. What are the Symptoms of Adult GH Deficiency (AGHD)?

- Decreased quantity and quality of life.
- Chronic fatigue.
- Decreased confidence and optimism.
- Lack of drive and vigor.
- Decreased muscle tone, increased droopiness.
- Loss of concentration.
- Sarcopenia (loss of muscle mass).[2]
- Anxiety.
- Sexual function disorders.
- Social isolation.
- Decreased slow wave sleep.[3]
- Loss of strength.
- Osteopenia, osteoporosis (loss of bone density).
- Glucose intolerance.
- Increased skin wrinkling and decreased skin thickness.
- Depressed mood.
- Increased total and intra-abdominal fat.
- Atherosclerosis.
- Increased fragility of skin and blood vessels.
- Loss of endurance.
- Reduced immunity and healing.
- Loss of exercise capacity.
- Increased total cholesterol, LDL cholesterol, and apolipoprotein B.

4. Most Physicians Won't Treat GH Levels That Aren't Really, Really Low.

MOST PHYSICIANS TREAT ONLY SEVERE HORMONAL DEFICIENCIES, not the more common hormonal deficiencies that occur as we age. Anti-aging physicians treat *all* low hormone levels, no matter how severe. Anti-aging physicians treat mild, moderate and extreme deficiencies of GH.

If Growth Hormone is below lab reference values, it is diagnostic of Adult GH Deficiency (AGHD), a rare disorder. This is what most physicians *will* treat. The diagnosis of Adult GH Deficiency is made by IGF-1 levels or urinary GH levels below lab reference values[4] and poor response to GHRH.

"Subclinical" decrease in hormone levels means that hormone levels have dropped to pathologically low levels, but not enough to meet the diagnostic criteria of AGHD and for the physician to recommend hormonal supplementation.

This does not mean that you would not benefit from treatment, just that most doctors will not treat you. Because this drop is pathological (below what the individual needs for good health), it will drift down to levels diagnostic of AGHD if we wait long enough. During this subclinical drop, the bones demineralize, muscle mass fades away, the immune system weakens, and vitality is low.

Traditional doctors would want to wait until the problem was really, really bad, i.e., extremely GH-deficient. By then, you would have deteriorated so much that it would be very difficult to lose all of the fat that you gained, and to gain back all of the muscle mass and bone density that you lost as your GH levels dropped to the point where you met their strict definition of GH deficiency.

If a GH decrease is "subclinical," your GH is within normal laboratory limits, but there is pathology present and it will end up in AGHD. Subclinical GH decrease produces a mild to moderate frailty syndrome. Anti-aging physicians believe that subclinical low levels of GH *should* be treated. One or five or ten years from now, it will become true GH *deficiency (AGHD)*, as your GH is headed down, down, down. By that time, your health will have deteriorated significantly.

If GH is suboptimal, it is within normal lab limits, but it isn't the progressive pathology that will lead to AGHD. If GH is drifting down from age, poor health, but not a pathological depression—it is called GH *insufficiency*. These suboptimal levels of GH mean that

GH is low for you for optimal health. GH levels may be age-appropriate, meaning you have declining hormone levels as you get older and wear out. But if you had higher, optimal levels, you would be more vital, live longer, age less quickly, build stronger bones and more muscle, and lose fat. Anti-aging physicians treat *all* low hormone levels, no matter how severe.

By the strictest definition, any person with IGF-1 levels less than 100 mcg/ml is GH-deficient (AGHD). But many anti-aging experts use anything less than 350 mcg/ml as GH-deficient.

If GH levels are subclinically depressed, treatment can be of great benefit to your health and well-being. Your health would significantly improve if GH were optimized. Many anti-aging experts recommend that you restore GH hormone levels to those of a healthy 32-year old for optimal health.

As we age, *most of us in the U.S.* have levels of GH that are too low for optimal health. Aboriginal cultures that live as hunter-gatherers in an environment without toxic pollution don't have these problems.

Check GH levels along with all of the other hormones that decline as we age. It's easy to overlook low GH.

5. Subclinical GH May Be Confused with Other Hormone Deficiencies.

SUBCLINICAL GH IS DIFFICULT TO DIAGNOSE because the loss of muscle mass, bone mass, and immune dysfunction looks much like other hormone deficiencies and aging. Subclinical GH may be overlooked when dealing with andropause, menopause, or thyroid problems.

Low testosterone symptoms (loss of muscle mass and bone density) are very similar to low GH symptoms. Andropause (male menopause) is characterized by low testosterone. Doctors call this condition "hypogonadism." But low testosterone may not be the only hormone deficiency of andropause. GH levels should also be considered.

The same goes for menopausal females. Estrogen and progesterone deficiencies in menopause cause symptoms very similar to GH deficiency—weight gain and Osteopenia.

Hypothyroidism causes similar symptoms to those of low GH. Low thyroid hormone levels cause deficient metabolism, cognition decline, and mood disorders, the same symptoms of deficient GH.

6. Why Treat GH Deficiency/Subclinical Depression/Suboptimal GH levels?

- GH treatment effectively treats the frailty syndrome of AGHD by increasing muscle mass, bone mass and density, cardiovascular strength, improved tissue strength, size and health of organs, and increased longevity.

- Data from extensive research shows increased energy, endurance, vitality, libido, and happiness when GH insufficiency is treated.

- Replacing GH improves inflammation, brain function,[5] bone density, atherosclerosis, heart function and strength,[6][7][8] immune system,[9] body composition, exercise capacity, wound healing, well-being, quality of life, and appearance.

- Treatment with GH decreases inflammatory chemicals (C-reactive protein) and improves insulin resistance.[10]

- GH has been associated with improvement in some cases of intractable diseases of aging: a variety of heart diseases, osteoporosis, Parkinson's disease, and diabetes.

- GH combined with the standard treatment for heart failure produces improvement in circulation and heart strength.

- Osteoporosis decreases 3-5% per year as GH and IGF-1 stimulate bone-building cells.

- AIDS patients benefit with increased muscle building as well as improved absorption of nutrients from the GI tract.

- Patients with Crohn's disease and ulcerative colitis have benefited, as well as leaky-gut syndrome patients. The law 333E specifically allows the use of GH in short-bowel syndrome and AIDS.

All of these benefits are ample reasons to keep GH levels within the normal range. This is real health insurance. Insure that you remain healthy into old age by keeping important hormones like GH at optimum levels.

Now let's see how GH helps all of the other hormones to do their job better. Then we will learn how to find out if *your* GH levels are too low.

7. GH Interacts with Every Other Hormone.

GH MAKES ALL THE OTHER HORMONES WORK by "up-regulating" the receptors. GH increases the number of receptors on the cells for estrogen, progesterone, pregnenolone, and every other hormone.[11] GH is like the doorman who opens the doors on the cells so that the other hormones can come in and do their jobs.

Need for replacement of other hormones may be eliminated or reduced when replacing growth hormone.[12] Estrogen and testosterone increase GH and GH increases estrogen and testosterone.

If GH is suboptimal or deficient, and you are *not* replacing it, the effect of replacing other hormones will be significantly less effective. If you add it on after you have begun other hormones, you may find that the effects of the other hormones may increase and you will have to decrease the other hormones.

It is best to begin replacing GH at the same time as beginning replacement of the other hormones in GH-insufficient people.

Women require higher doses, the elderly require lower doses.

8. How Do You Know if Your Own Levels of Growth Hormone are Inadequate?

You need to see your doctor and get tested.

IGF-1 is a growth factor. It stands for Insulin Growth Factor-1. This is the test that measures GH levels.

GH, itself, is not what produces the increase in muscle mass, bone mass, and fat loss. GH stimulates the production of *growth factors* in the tissues that actually stimulate the tissues to grow and repair.

Measuring IGF-1 is the most accurate assessment of GH levels. IGF-1 is the most prominent of these growth factors.

GH levels fluctuate very rapidly. Therefore your doctor usually checks IGF-1 levels, which are much more stable, or urinary GH levels.

Your doctor may also recommend a GH stimulation test, where Growth Hormone Releasing Hormone (GHRH) is injected and the response of the pituitary to this hypothalamic-releasing hormone is measured.

Evaluation and Treatment Lab: These are the labs that are recommended.

Hormone replacement must be monitored.
- Get a serum IGF-1, IGFBP3, and urine GH.[13]
- Free testosterone and DH-testosterone.
- DHEA-S.
- Females: E1 (estrone), E2 (estradiol), progesterone.
- Males: E1, E2, testosterone, zinc.

If you find out that your GH is low, there are some things that you should consider before jumping right in and treating it.

9. Before You Begin Treatment

You must be very careful before you begin to use supplements that raise your body's levels of Growth Hormone. Some of these supplements increase your risk for getting cancer or may strain your heart.

I got skin cancer from using a GH stimulant. When I hit menopause, I felt terrible. In a misguided attempt to bring my energy back, I started to take a Growth Hormone treatment.

It made me feel great! But after only two weeks of use, a deadly skin cancer, squamous cell carcinoma, began to grow out of the end of my nose.

Four thousand dollars and a dreadful operation later, the cancer was gone. I was left with a scar on my nose as the only evidence of the ordeal. I learned the hard way not to mess around with Growth Hormone stimulators.

Some of these supplements can kill you. I was lucky that this was a visible cancer. If dormant cancer cells had been in a more hidden place, the GH treatment could have promoted them to grow into a life-threatening illness that could have killed me before I even knew what had happened. Because I could see the tumor immediately as it formed, I was able to get the treatment that saved my life. The surgeon removed every cancer cell from the end of my nose immediately.

Some of my friends weren't so lucky. They no longer walk with us on this earth because of their use of steroids like this.

GH has great potential benefit and great risk. Use it under the supervision of your doctor and understand the risk you are taking.

Be sure that DHEA levels are adequate before using GH. GH stimulates the production of growth factors in the tissues, especially IGF-1 (insulin-like growth factor 1) in the liver. GH and DHEA *both* raise levels of IGF-1, an anabolic hormone. DHEA replaced transdermally is usually the most effective route.

GH receptor resistance or insensitivity may be caused by toxicity and may contribute to GH deficiency. Address toxicity by cleansing.[14] Nothing you do to increase your GH will work when toxicity is blocking the cell receptors (the doors on the cells that allow the hormones to enter). Please read chapter 27 of my book, Secrets about Bioidentical Hormones.[15] It details how to remove toxicity from your body.

Next we will explore how to treat low GH naturally. Then we will move on to the more potent treatment modalities.

10. How Can I Raise my GH Naturally?

FOR SUBCLINICAL AND SUBOPTIMAL GH levels, first use diet, exercise, vitamins, anti-oxidants, herbs, homeopathics, and omega-3's.

GH rises with intense physical activity, such as weight-lifting or interval training, and when eating plenty of protein or fasting. Zinc is required for GH to work. Symptoms of zinc deficiency are very similar to GH deficiency—poor wound healing, immunosuppression, impaired protein synthesis and decreased hormone levels. Niacinamide (B-3) increases GH, as well as calcium. Effective herbal GH stimulants include Maca, Mucuna Pruriens, and Tribulus Terrestis.

Over-the-counter oral GH secretagogues. The safest and most natural treatment is the stimulation of growth-hormone releasing hormone (GHRH) from the hypothalamus and GH from the pituitary.[16]

The hypothalamus is a gland in the brain that controls all of the hormones in the body. If the hypothalamus has been injured in a brain injury, GH levels may drop (along with other hormones). Anything that can help to heal the hypothalamus may help impaired GH production.

Homeopathics may be effective for some people. CranialSacral Therapy may help also.

The hippocampus controls the hypothalamus. It may deteriorate, especially as the result of chronic stress or PTSD. The adrenal adaptogens are the best treatment for the degeneration of the hippocampus. See my book, <u>Secrets about Bioidentical Hormones</u>,[17] to learn about the adrenal adaptogens.

Over-the-counter oral GH secretagogues include L-arginine, L-glutamine, L-ornithine, ornithine alpha-ketoglutarate (OKG), L-dopa, glycine, GABA, and B-6.

GH Production is Stimulated By:

- **Growth hormone releasing hormone (GHRH)** from the hypothalamus.

- **Ghrelin** (sGHS-receptors). Secretagogues (discussed below) work through the Ghrelin and HGH releasing receptors.

- **Sleep**--GH is normally produced while we sleep. Therefore, sleep disturbances of a pathological nature can impair GH production and release. Melatonin supplementation may increase sleep. Get to bed early and make an effort to get plenty of sleep. Without restorative sleep, Growth Hormone (GH) production is impaired. Without GH, your tissues begin to break down. Sleep disruption also interferes with nerve cell renewal causing major depression.[18]

- **Intense aerobic activity.** Work out regularly and increase your ability to run, walk, bike, swim, and do other aerobic activities for longer periods of time. Work up to an hour three or more days each week.

- **Dietary protein** (ornithine, pyroglutamine, arginine, and alpha-ketoglutarate) causes stimulation of receptors. Supplement with protein powders. At every meal, eat a wide variety of meats, fish, and eggs, if no allergies exist.

- **Estradiol** in women increases HGH release from the pituitary,[19] the gland that releases GH. Estradiol is the estrogen that is secreted by women in their reproductive years. Menopausal women can raise their GH levels by using supplemental Estradiol. Estradiol is available only by prescription. Please read my books about bioidentical hormones for complete information about using estradiol. [20,21]

- **Arginine** (via suppression of somatostatin, also called HGH-inhibiting hormone). This is a supplement that can be found in health food stores.[22]

- **Stress reduction.** As stress increases, GH levels drop.

11. Treatment

Where can I find a doctor who will treat low GH levels? Because of strict laws, few doctors will treat the GH decline associated with aging and even fewer will be willing to optimize GH. Let's look at the law.

333E is the law passed in 1988 regulating the use of GH. This law prohibits the use of GH for conditions outside its narrow parameters. The law allows the use of GH for: (1) wasting syndrome of AIDS, (2) short bowel syndrome, and (3) Adult GH *Deficiency* (AGHD). AGHD is a rare condition. But the subclinical insufficiency or suboptimal levels often associated with aging are very common. The off-label use of HGH and IGF-1 are not allowed in the U.S. AGHD must be diagnosed by an abnormal pituitary response to the injection of GHRH.

Your best bet for getting treated is from an anti-aging physician. Many may be found through these groups:

American Academy of Anti-Aging Medicine (A4M)
888-997-0112   http://www.worldhealth.net/

American College for Advancement in Medicine (ACAM)
800-532-3688   http://www.acamnet.org

12. Treatment Modalities:

START WITH THE SAFEST METHODS OF TREATMENT. The following treatment modalities are listed in increasing order of effectiveness, but decreasing order of safety in terms of their ability to stimulate an existing cancer tumor, no matter how small.[23] You must be more careful as you move down this list. Over-zealous body-builders and others using the strongest GH stimulators are at great risk for developing life-threatening illness.

The bottom line: Don't mess around with supplements designed to increase GH. See an anti-aging doctor and follow his or her advice to take the supplements *only* when your own GH is low.

1. **Hypothalamic peptides and GH stimulants** from amino acids and plant extracts are higher in potency with possible increased side effects when compared to the natural treatments listed in Chapter 10. To order, call Guy (that's his name) at Bodyworx. His number is (877) 663-3438.

   Symbiotropin®: is a *non-prescription* herbal-based formula that treats decreased GH in several ways.
   - Secretagogues (stimulate GH release).
   - Receptor-site modulators (plant-based) to improve GH & IGF-1 receptor sensitivity.

- Insulin modulators.
- Liver enzyme enhancers.

Meditropin®: is a stronger, second-generation, oral secretagogue, *available only through physicians.* Meditropin stimulates releasing hormones from the hypothalamus and GH from the pituitary. It uses:
- Hypothalamic-stimulating peptides (porcine glandular products).
- Protein growth factors from colostrum (first milk).
- The other factors that are found in Symbiotropin.

Take secretagogues on a completely empty stomach. Insulin counteracts the actions of IGF-1, so the maximum value of any GH increase is attained by keeping insulin levels low. The majority of GH is secreted during the night, so secretagogues are taken at bedtime or during the night, although morning doses work well and are often included.

2. **Injectable secretagogues (unavailable for *human* use in the U.S.).** The next mode of treatment which is more effective, with more possible side effects, is the stimulation of receptors in the hypothalamus and pituitary with injectable secretagogues. They are sold on the internet (for investigational use) without a prescription.

Primary advantages of the injectable secretagogues are:

- They stimulate the production and release of hypothalamic and pituitary hormones.
- They cause a more natural, pulsatile release of GH.
- They cost less than GHRH or GH injections.
- They may have protective effects on the neurons in the central nervous system.

GH-releasing peptides-6 (GHRP-6) and Hexarelin release GH by:
- Amplifying the GHRH signal in the hypothalamus.
- Inhibiting GH inhibiting hormone (GHIH or Somatostatin), in the hypothalamus.
- Direct stimulation of the anterior pituitary release of GH.

The primary adverse side effect of GHRP-6 (Growth Hormone Releasing Peptide-6) is increased appetite and resulting weight gain because it activates Ghrelin receptor sites in the hypothalamus. Hexarelin does not increase appetite. If you have been using HGHr or IGF-1 injections, it is particularly advantageous to use GHRP-6 or GHRH to stimulate the pituitary and hypothalamic atrophy that results from the injections.

3. GHRH injections. The next treatment level, which is more effective and expensive, is GH Releasing

Hormone (**Sermorelin**). You need a prescription to get it.

The primary advantages of GHRH injections are their ability to stimulate the body's production and release of hypothalamic and pituitary hormones, and more natural pulsatile release of hormones.

Sermorelin is the first 29 amino acids of GH. This amino acid sequence is what stimulates the pituitary to release growth hormone. Because of the intact negative feedback to the hypothalamus and release of somatostatin (GH-inhibiting hormone), GH overdose is avoided. Also it is not prohibited by federal law for off-label use, as HGH is.

Sermorelin produces less tissue down-regulation and has more normal pulsatile regulation than injectable HGH because of hypothalamic feedback.

4. **Injectable Human Growth Hormone (HGH).** HGHr (recombinant HGH) is the most effective treatment of GH deficiency with the highest side effect profile. It is very expensive and available only by prescription.

The primary advantages of HGHr are the ability to achieve high hormone levels.

One of the biggest downsides of injectable HGH is the profound atrophy that occurs in the body's natural production system for GH, and GH-receptor down-regulation. The more you take and the longer you take it, the less effective it becomes. When you stop taking it, your muscles will lose tone rapidly, and you will be transiently GH-deficient until your own GH system comes back on line.

The primary disadvantages are the cost, atrophy in the hypothalamus and pituitary, receptor down-regulation, and the ability to achieve pathologically high GH levels, with its multitude of dangers and side effects.

HGHr produces tissue down-regulation because of the high levels and the lack of a normal, pulsatile release.

There are four primary side effects to look out for, "PAGE": paresthesias, arthralgias, glucose and insulin getting worse instead of better, and edema.

HGH injections may produce diabetes, insulin resistance with hypoglycemia and hyperglycemia, carpal tunnel syndrome, aching joints, hypotension and hypertension, cardiovascular disease and heart failure, uncontrolled bleeding, ketogenesis, GI disturbance, gynecomastia, allergic response, and iatrogenic acromegaly (thickening of bones of jaw, fingers, and toes).

There is extensive data to suggest that *HGH does not cause cancer, but could stimulate the growth of existing neoplasms, even microscopic.*

Contraindications include uncompensated diabetes mellitus, heart failure, smoking, and known or unknown malignant tumors.[24]

5. **Long-chain IGF-1 injections** are available outside the U.S. (on the internet) and are highly effective, but *the most dangerous* of all treatment modalities. IGF-1 is likely to greatly facilitate the growth of existing tumors, even if microscopic. It is not proven to induce cancer, but the studies are incomplete.

Increlix is IGF-1 that is now available by prescription. However, the indications are very restricted and off-label use is discouraged.

6. **Tissue Growth factors.** Many other tissue growth factors produced in the body by GH are becoming available online. These are becoming prominent in the body-building industry. These are not approved for use in the U.S. or generally available. These growth factors are incredibly powerful and little is know about their use.

REFERENCES

[1] Besson A, Salemi S, Gallati S, Jenal A, Horn R, Mullis PS, Mullis PE. Reduced longevity in untreated patients with isolated growth hormone deficiency. *J Clin Endocrinol Metab. 2003 Aug;88(8):3664-7.*

[2] Visser M, Pahor M, Taaffe DR, Goodpaster BH, Simonsick EM, Newman AB, Nevitt M, Harris TB. Relationship of interleukin-6 and tumor necrosis factor-alpha with muscle mass and muscle strength in elderly men and women: the Health ABC Study. *J Gerontol A Biol Sci Med Sci. 2002 May;57(5):M326-32.*

[3] Van Cauter E, Leproult R, Plat L. Age-related changes in slow wave sleep and REM sleep and relationship with growth hormone and cortisol levels in healthy men. *JAMA. 2000 Aug 16;284(7):861-8.*

[4] Biller BM, Samuels MH, Agar A, Cook DM, Arafat BM, Binnert V, Stavros S, Kleinberg DL, Chapman JJ, Hartman ML. Sensitivity and specificity of six tests for the diagnosis of adult GH deficiency. *J Clinic Endocrinology Metabolism 2002; 87(5):2067-79.*

[5] Cranston, IC, Marsden PK et al. Effects of HGH replacement on cerebral metabolism in adults with growth hormone deficiency. *Growth Hormone and IGF Research 1998 UMDS St Thomas Hospital, London, UK.*

[6] Colao A, Di Somma C, Savanelli MC, De Leo M, Lombardi G. Beginning to end: cardiovascular implications of growth hormone (GH) deficiency and GH therapy. *Growth Horm IGF Res. 2006 Jul;16 Suppl A:S41-8.*

[7] Oflaz H, Sen F, Elitok A, Cimen AO, Onur I, Kasikcioglu E, Korkmaz S, Demirturk M, Kutluturk F, Pamukcu B, Ozbey N. Coronary flow reserve is impaired in patients with adult growth hormone (GH) deficiency. *Clin Endocrinol (Oxf). 2007 Apr;66(4):524-9.*

[8] Sesmilo G, Biller BM, Llevadot J, Hayden D, Hanson G, Rifai N, Klibanski A. Effects of growth hormone administration on inflammatory and other cardiovascular risk markers in men with growth hormone deficiency. A randomized, controlled clinical trial. *Ann Intern Med. 2000 Jul 18;133(2):111-22.*

[9] Gelato, MC. Aging and immune function: a possible role for growth hormone. *Horm Res 1996; 45(1-2)46-9.*

[10] Andreassen M, Vestergaard H, Kristensen LØ.. Concentrations of the acute phase reactants high-sensitive C-reactive protein and YKL-40 and of interleukin-6 before and after treatment in patients with

acromegaly and growth hormone deficiency. *Clin Endocrinol (Oxf). 2007 Dec;67(6):909-16.*

[11] Björntorp P. Growth hormone, insulin-like growth factor-I and lipid metabolism: interactions with sex steroids. *Horm Res. 1996;46(4-5):188-91.*

[12] Meinhardt UJ, Ho KK. Modulation of growth hormone action by sex steroids. *Clin Endocrinol (Oxf). 2006 Oct;65(4):413-22.*

[13] Clemmons, DR. Commercial assays available for insulin-like growth factor I and their use in diagnosing growth hormone deficiency. *Horm Res. 2001; 55 Suppl 2:73-9.*

[14] Wright YL. *Secrets about Bioidentical Hormones to Lose Fat and Prevent Cancer, Heart Disease, Menopause, and Andropause, by Optimizing Adrenals, Thyroid, Estrogen, Progesterone, Testosterone, and Growth Hormone!* Lulu.com. December 18, 2010.

[15] Wright YL. *Secrets about Bioidentical Hormones to Lose Fat and Prevent Cancer, Heart Disease, Menopause, and Andropause, by Optimizing Adrenals, Thyroid, Estrogen, Progesterone, Testosterone, and Growth Hormone!* Lulu.com. December 18, 2010. p.66

[16] Peñalva A, Carballo A, Pombo M, Casanueva FF, Dieguez C. Effect of growth hormone (GH)-releasing hormone (GHRH), atropine, pyridostigmine, or hypoglycemia on GHRP-6-induced GH secretion in man. *J Clin Endocrinol Metab. 1993 Jan;76(1):168-71.*

[17] Wright YL. *Secrets about Bioidentical Hormones to Lose Fat and Prevent Cancer, Heart Disease, Menopause, and Andropause, by Optimizing Adrenals, Thyroid, Estrogen, Progesterone, Testosterone, and Growth Hormone!* Lulu.com. December 18, 2010. p.48

[18] Myint AM, Kim YK. Cytokine-serotonin interaction through IDO: a neurodegeneration hypothesis of depression. *Med Hypotheses. 2003 Nov-Dec;61(5-6):519-25.*

[19] Trudeau VL, Somoza GM, Nahorniak CS, Peter RE. Interactions of estradiol with gonadotropin-releasing hormone and thyrotropin-releasing hormone in the control of growth hormone secretion in the goldfish. *Neuroendocrinology. 1992Oct;56(4):483-90.*

[20] Wright YL. *Secrets about Bioidentical Hormones to Lose Fat and Prevent Cancer, Heart Disease, Menopause, and Andropause, by Optimizing Adrenals, Thyroid, Estrogen, Progesterone, Testosterone, and Growth Hormone!* Lulu.com. December 18, 2010.

[21] Wright YL. *Bioidentical Hormones Mady Easy!* Lulu.com. 2011.

[22] Alba-Roth J, Müller OA, Schopohl J, von Werder K. Arginine

stimulates growth hormone secretion by suppressing endogenous somatostatin secretion. *J Clin Endocrinol Metab. 1988 Dec;67(6):1186-9.*

[23] Jenkins PJ, Mukherjee A, Shalet SM. Does growth hormone cause cancer? *Clin Endocrinol (Oxf). 2006 Feb;64(2):115-21.*

[24] Darzy KH, Shalet SM. Pathophysiology of radiation-induced growth hormone deficiency: efficacy and safety of GH replacement. *Growth Horm IGF Res. 2006; 16 Suppl A: S30-40.*

INDEX

abdominal fat, 8
aerobic, 22
AIDS, 14, 23
anabolic, 19
appetite, 26
body composition, 13
bone, 7, 8, 28
cancer, 24, 29
cardiovascular, 28, 30
chemicals, 13
cholesterol, 8
colitis, 14
cortisol, 30
C-reactive protein, 13
Crohn's, 14
depression, 22
DHEA, 17, 19
diabetes, 13, 28, 29
E2, 17
Estradiol, 22
estrogen, 15
exercise, 8, 13
fatigue, 8
GABA, 21
GH, 7, 8, 9 15, 17, 19, 20, 21, 23, 24, 25, 26, 27, 30
GH deficiency, 9, 13, 19, 20, 23
GH insufficiency, 11
ghrelin, 21
GHRH injections, 26
GHRP-6, 26
glucose, 28
gut, 14
heart, 13, 28, 29
heart diseases, 13
Hexarelin, 26
HGH, 21, 22, 23, 27, 28, 30
hypertension, 28
Hypothalamic peptides, 24
hypothalamus, 20, 21, 25, 26, 27, 28
iatrogenic, 28

IGF-1, 9, 14, 17, 19, 23, 24, 25, 26, 29
immune system, 7, 8, 13
Increlix, 29
inflammation, 13, 30
Injectable Human Growth Hormone, 27
insulin, 13, 19, 25, 28
insulin resistance, 13, 28
libido, 13
liver, 7, 19
Long-chain, 29
metabolism, 30
mood, 8
muscle mass, 7, 8, 30
omega-3, 20
Osteopenia, 8
Osteoporosis, 8, 13, 14
Parkinson's, 13
physical activity, 20
pituitary, 20, 23, 25, 26, 27, 28
pregnenolone, 15
progesterone, 15, 17
protein, 20, 22
receptor resistance, 19
receptor sites, 26
receptors, 15, 21, 22, 25
Sarcopenia, 8
secretagogues, 21, 24, 25
skin, 8
sleep, 8, 21, 22, 30
smoking, 29
stimulants, 20, 24
testosterone, 15, 17
toxicity, 19
tumor, 24, 30
urine, 17
vitality, 13
weight, 20, 26
weight gain, 26
wrinkling, 8

Made in the USA
Lexington, KY
23 August 2014